ULTIMATE GUIDE TO MAKING

LIVE ORGANIC KEFIR

HOW TO ENSURE HIGHEST COUNT

OF PROBIOTICS FOR MAXIMUM

HEALTH BENEFITS

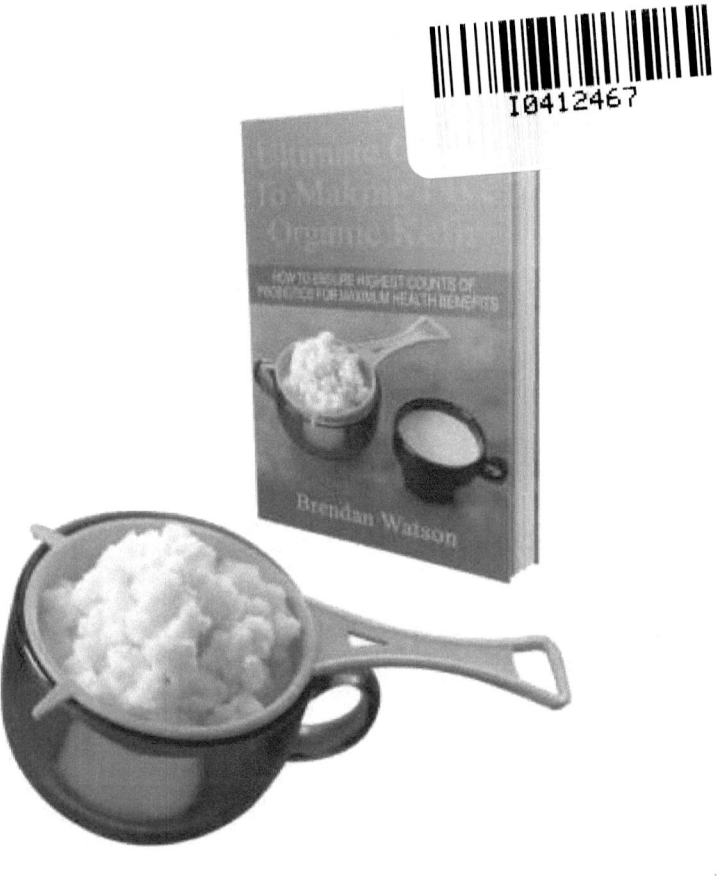

document is not allowed unless with written permission from the publisher. All rights reserved.

The information provided herein is stated to be truthful and consistent, in that any liability, in terms of inattention or otherwise, by any usage or abuse of any policies, processes, or directions contained within is the solitary and utter responsibility of the recipient reader. Under no circumstances will any legal responsibility or blame be held against the publisher for any reparation, damages, or monetary loss due to the information herein, either directly or indirectly.

Professional or Medical Advice Disclaimer

The purpose of this book is for educational and informational purposes only and is made available to you as self-educational materials and tools for your own use. All materials and information are to educate, inform and inspire you to heal. The author does not provide health care, medical or nutritional therapy services and will not diagnose, prevent, treat, or cure in any manner whatsoever any disease, condition or other physical or mental ailment of the human body. The information in or through this book is not intended to replace a one-on-one relationship with a qualified healthcare professional. As such, it is not intended as a substitute for the advice provided by your physician or other healthcare providers, and it is not intended as medical advice, diagnosis, or treatment. This book does not take the place of your doctor, licensed dietician, nutritionist, psychologist, nurse, mental health provider, physician's assistant or any other licensed or registered health care professional.

Table of Contents

INTRODUCTION

Ultimate Guide to Making Live Organic Kefir at Home - How to Ensure Highest Count of Probiotics For Maximum Health Benefits

Kefir has gained more popularity in recent years. Partly due to increased gut related illness from greater antibiotic uses.

This book contains proven steps and strategies to maximize the health benefits by consuming trillions of probiotics or the good/beneficial bacteria that are fresh and homemade. This will save you literally thousands of dollars in purchasing expired, near expired probiotic pills. Did you know that probiotic numbers you see on the bottle are at the time they were tested and manufactured not the time you consume them! The actual probiotics in those bottles may be next to zero when you consume them. The numbers you see on the probiotics bottle are NOT the number of live probiotics that you are consuming!!

This is because many probiotics die well before you ever get benefit from them. Some bacteria require refrigeration; even though you see them in the refrigeration shelves at your retail store it does not mean that they were in refrigeration the entire time! Shelves at grocery stores are just a big showcase! Do you know if the probiotic bottles were actually delivered to that store in a refrigerated truck? Even if they were transited in a refrigerated truck, there are too many variables you cannot be certain of. For example, what was the time they were sitting at the dock of the warehouse before they were loaded onto the truck? At delivery, how long were they stored in back of the warehouse before they were stocked? How many pit stops did the truck make? If the truck made pit stop, did the refrigeration turn off? If employees were busy at delivery, when did they have time to stock them? Sometimes this process takes minutes; other times hours and days based on employee hours, managers priorities, etc. During this idle time millions of beneficial bacteria are dying inside the capsule.

This is why I recommend making your own probiotics and consuming fresh batches daily. This way you take out all the variables, all the marketing gimmicks and you know what you are getting.

This book's objective is for you to learn how to maximize beneficial bacteria delivered to you; and the only tangible way to ensure this is by consuming

FRESH batches of probiotics you made at home. This way you are in full control of what you are consuming. If something is fermented and it is changing its composition, you know it is alive! As the old saying goes "If you want it done right, do it yourself!"

Kefir has been around for thousands of years. If you follow the procedures in this book, you will be consuming not billions but trillions of probiotics daily. It is more potent than pills, since it has thriving probiotics that are made the same day you consume the product, not something that has been sitting on the shelves for months or at times years without any entity regulating them! FDA does not regulate probiotics, neither does any other agency at the time of publishing this book.

Once you purchase these grains you do not need to repurchase them, as long as you can manage them.

A few dollars will go a long way!

CHAPTER 1: WHAT IS KEFIR?

Approximately 3,000 years ago, researchers found out that kefir grains were originated somewhere near Caucasus Mountains (north of Turkey/Iran/Armenia). It was the result of keeping milk pasteurized.

It was believed that the region between the Black and Caspian Seas in Eurasia (located between Russia and Asia) was accidentally discovered by Edward Kern, a German Naturalist, in the Caucasus Mountains. He told St. Petersburg's Botanic Society that he had discovered an unusual kind of beverage, and that he noticed how people living in the area were pretty healthy and had high life expectancy. Of course, there are many reasons for this, not just kefir. However, since then, a lot of research has been going into determining what the locals were consuming and their lifestyle. This was followed by many scientists who tested kefir in the Caucasus mountains, where there was poor sanitary condition, but people lived long lives. In further tests scientists were said to inject bacteria such as e. coli and h. pylori into the kefir drink, but the probiotics crowded out the harmful bacteria and destroyed them! They found this drink to not only rid the harmful bacteria but stimulate immune system.

The term "Kefir" was concocted by the Turks and Russians around the same time, 3,000 years ago. As the benefits of kefir started to grow in the middle east, different recipes of kefir started to emerge. They ranged from water kefir, or one that is made with coconut or sugar-flavored water, but without any dairy, however the most popular was still milk kefir.

Kefir is a healthy alternative to milk. It has a creamy consistency that can taste like buttermilk or sour cream and can also be flavored so it would not taste too tangy. It is made by combining kefir grains with cow, goat, or sheep's milk, and fermenting them to create a drink loaded with probiotics.

There are many flavorings and scents added to kefir drinks. It also serves as an alternative to fruit juices or soda and can be mixed with a whole lot of ingredients to create flavorful appetizing and nutritious drink. You may see familiar drinks on the market such as "kombucha" which are clearer than milk kefir. There are hundreds of other recipes for making kefir on the market today. This is not a recipe book, but we will deep dive into making the best, potent kefir from grains and milk. As you feel comfortable you can experiment with other recipes, based on the type of taste and flavoring you like.

KEFIR GRAINS

No matter what type of kefir you like to make, they are all initially made from kefir grains.

These grains are white in color, sometimes a little yellow has rough gelatinous feel to it, like little cauliflowers. They do come in different shapes and sizes, sometimes are plumped up and other times flat. They tend to be a little slimy. These are not typical grains you can manufacture by adding different ingredients or harvest at a farm. These kefir grains survive, grow, and replicate mostly on lactose (type of sugar found in milk and dairy) and the right environment. Fermentation takes place, where the lactose from milk is converted to carbon dioxide and lactic acid.

These grains naturally contain beneficial bacteria/probiotics, other live microorganisms such as yeast and even some enzymes that strengthen the digestive system. These beneficial microorganisms help crowd out or out-compete the pathogenic organisms inside your gut.

STRAINS COMMONLY FOUND IN KEFIR:

- ✓ Lactobacilli

- ✓ Leuconostoc

- ✓ Acetobacter Aceti

- ✓ Streptococci

- ✓ Lactococci

- ✓ Enterococci

- ✓ Other Bacteria (Bacillus, Bacillus Subtilis, etc.)

I will teach you how to add other probiotics into your kefir, so you are not dependent on store bought pills-Keep Reading!

CHAPTER 2: WHAT ARE THE BENEFITS OF CONSUMING KEFIR PROBIOTICS?

Most fermented food such as yogurt contain beneficial bacteria, however kefir has more than one branch of good bacteria in it—and those branches even contain various strains of good bacteria, too, which means that it truly is one of the best probiotics you can consume. Kefir is also full of enzymes, nutrients that balance your inner gut ecosystem that strengthens immunity.

Yogurt Vs. Kefir

The advantages to kefir over yogurt:

- Kefir is known to colonize more effectively than yogurt, so that probiotics do not pass through your gut, but actually start to reproduce. This also depends on the strains, prebiotics and fiber called inulin.

- You are not limited to strains that are in yogurt, you can add, modify, and control strains in your kefir. Your body may do well with some strains over others. I will show you how you can add additional strains to your kefir batches in later chapter.

- Concentration of probiotics in your kefir can far outweigh few probiotics that are found in store bought yogurt. You would need to eat gallons of yogurt what can be found in glass of kefir drink.

- Drinking and flavoring kefir drink is more palatable than eating yogurt.

- You do not need to continuously go to store to purchase company manufactured yogurt which sometimes have preservatives and added sugar for flavoring.

- Flavored yogurts are even worse, they are loaded with refined sugar and preservatives, pectin, dextrose, gum. Once you are adding sugar, you are actually taking out the benefits from probiotics and this fosters growth of candida.

Milk Kefir Vs. Water Kefir

If you are vegan or lactose intolerant (even though milk kefir is quite easy to digest, unlike other milk products), you can opt to make water kefir. Some enjoy the taste of water kefir more than milk kefir. Be sure to use non-chlorinated water (as chlorine will kill of some of the bacteria), you can also use soda stream to add some fizz in your drink, along with cucumber, lemon and stevia would make great refreshing summertime drink. Water kefir has the same probiotics and mineral effect but is less bulky.

Water Kefir Tips-2 Ingredients to Watch Out For

This is not a recipe book, so I don't want to list bunch of recipes here, however this book was written to show you how to make ultimate milk kefir from kefir grains (Chapter 6). However lately much has been said about water kefir. I would like to keep the following in mind if you plan to make water kefir.

Best Types of Sugar in Water Kefir

If you use water kefir, you will want to add taste to this. Unfortunately, most of the time adding taste means adding sugar. If you are using kefir to restore gut flora, sugar is the worst culprit. The kind of sugar you use may determine the number of probiotics that survive in your homemade kefir. Other sugar substitutes like xylitol and honey contain antimicrobial properties, which are great substitutes for sugar but may not be the best alternatives if your aim is for probiotics to grow!

RULE OF THUMB – LESS SUGAR THE BETTER!

That said, here is what you can use to sweeten Kefir:

ORGANIC CANE SUGAR

It is pretty sweet, but it is all natural, which means that it produces more enzymes that can give you the best kinds of probiotics.

PROCESSED WHITE CANE SUGAR

A pinch would be good already, but do not go any further than that because it will ruin the consistency and the nutritional make-up of Kefir.

FRUIT JUICE

Not only are they flavorful, but they will also make the kefir more colorful—so you could get kids and non-vegetarians to try them out, too. It also contains natural sugars that are not like the processed ones that you can find in the market. This makes probiotics prevalent in Kefir and will help you make sure that you are on to something good.

MOLASSES

What is great about molasses is that even if they are just by-products of sugar, you can expect that essential minerals are retained. It is best to mix molasses with organic cane sugar to make kefir that will yield the best results. It is tastier, too.

RAPADURA AND SUCANAT

Using these would make kefir that is darker than any other kind of kefir. What is good about them though is that they are forms of unrefined and whole cane sugar—so you would know that you would get a lot of benefits from them. Sucanat has molasses blended, taken out, and mixed back with it, while Rapadura has molasses intact, so it could produce results that are pretty sweet.

Best Type of Water in Water Kefir

WATER

And of course, water also plays a crucial role. What you must keep in mind is that it is best to stay away from water that is already contaminated with fluoride or chlorine (such as tap water), because this would not make your kefir nutritious at any rate. It can also hinder the growth of beneficial bacteria. Therefore, you have the following choices:

WELL WATER

For some reason, it is said that this is best for making kefir, presumably because it is all natural, it comes from the ground, and it has not been tampered with preservatives or techniques of any kind. This way, it would create a lot of probiotics and make Kefir healthy for you.

BOTTLED OR FILTERED WATER

If you are going to use filtered or bottled water for making kefir, it might be good if you could add some mineral drops just to make sure that what you will make will be in high-grade condition. Adding molasses when using filtered water can also be helpful.

COCONUT WATER

Coconut water is healthy, and it is also the reason why a lot of people choose it as an alternative to tap or mineral water. It can make Kefir effective and nutritious, so it is best that you choose this.

TAP WATER

And finally, if there are times when you feel like you cannot use other kinds of water, make sure that you treat it first so you can rid it of chlorine. First and foremost, use a filter to eliminate the chlorine and then put water in a blender and aerate it for around 12 hours so that you can be sure that the chlorine will evaporate, and so it will still be filled with the right minerals that you need and won't interfere with growth of your probiotics.

Health Benefits of Consuming Kefir

<u>DIGESTION</u>

Probiotics are essential because they AID IN HEALTH DIGESTION. Especially the ones found in nature, which protect from bile acids in the stomach and find their way to lower interesting to colonize. The right strains in proper amount have been known to treat Irritable Bowel Syndrome (IBS) and even assist in Crohn's disease. They have also been known to effectively reverse the effects of IBS and prevent further attacks in the future. If your digestion is not working nothing will, if you are not absorbing the right nutrients, it really does not matter what you are consuming. This is vital and kefir helps greatly in this process! It helps support your normal intestinal tract functions, promotes bowl movement. It also helps with other digestive disorders like gas, acid reflux and heartburn.

BOOSTS IMMUNITY

It is said that kefir is good for the body because of its multiprong approach that not only rids harmful bacteria with good ones but provides micronutrients. This helps regulate the body's immune system and improves resistance to many diseases.

DETOXIFY

It detoxifies the body. Kefir contains mutagens. Mutagens alter the DNA in such a way that it does not become susceptible to bad bacteria or diseases because it almost becomes one with the environment that the person is living in. This way, toxic chemicals are also prevented from entering the body—and you can't say that other types of probiotic-laded food products can do that! Kefirs are also responsible for diminishing aflatoxins that cause negative immune system reactions and allergies because of their high lactic acid content, which therefore make positive genetic expression possible!

LACTOSE INTOLERANCE

In many cases, kefir is tolerated well by people who are lactose intolerant. This is because bacteria break down the lactose in the milk yielding protein, vitamins, mineral and good fats. These broken-down nutrients are easier to digest and assimilate into your body. Some people hate milk because their bodies cannot take it in, or simply put, they are lactose-intolerant.

ALLERGIES & ASTHMA

It prevents allergies and asthma. Kefir can suppress the effects of immunoglobins and T-helper cells that cause respiratory inflammation. Therefore, the effects of asthma and allergies would be reduced because of it.

BONE DENSITY

One of the best things about Kefir is that it prevents the onset of Osteoporosis because it improves the body's absorption of important minerals such as magnesium and calcium, as well as Vitamin K2, Vitamin D, and calcium, as well.

OTHER BENEFITS

More so, recent studies have shown that Kefir may also help reduce weight, acne, prevent liver and Crohn's diseases, gum disease, cavities, kidney stones, cough, colds, flu, candida disease, and ulcers, and even autism (Even though I think autism claim may have been over simplified)

Probiotics in kefir are also known to kick out fungi, yeast, and bad bacteria from your gut.

Kefir is also rich in minerals and essential vitamins that the human body needs, such as Vitamin K-2, Vitamin B12, and Butyrate, B12, B1, pantothenic acid, folic acid, and biotin among others, which helps regulates blood flow, absorption which aids in cell and tissue regeneration!

Other less studied claims are that kefir can control high blood pressure, ADHD (promotes relaxing effect on the nervous system and even helps with restful sleep at night -mg+/Ca+), Also helps with ulcers, lung infection, eczema, kidney stones, and controls sugar that may help with diabetes.

A glass of kefir instead of sugary soda will go a long way to improving your health.

CHAPTER 3: KEFIR COMBATING HIDDEN CANDIDA & ANTIBIOTICS IN YOUR GUT (THAT YOU DON'T EVEN KNOW ABOUT) - HOW TO REBALANCE YOUR GUT

KNOW THE SOURCE

Kefir can definitely help you, granted you are being treated in the right condition. There is no way anyone can "fix" your specific ailment without knowing what is causing your ailment. You must know the source of your problem, know the cause. This requires a diagnosis of your condition. I am not a medical doctor to diagnose you, neither are lot false online promisers. Once you and/or your doctor diagnose your condition then you can begin to find a cure. Anyone who blindly promises you a fix and pushes a product/pill without diagnosing your problem is not out to help you; they are out to help themselves! Period!

However, it is well documented that kefir is known to help millions with imbalance of bacteria in their gut, which sometimes can lead to hosts of other diseases.

Ancient Greek physician Hippocrates nearly 2500 years ago stated, "All disease begins in the gut". Today, many alternative and even MDs are coming around to this concept. Consider "Leaky Gut Syndrome," where tiny holes in your gut allow toxins to permeate into your bloodstream. You can imagine if these toxins enter your bloodstream, how they can cause HAVOC on all parts of internal system. If your gut is out of balance, then you are out of balance!

It is not that kefir directly cures everything. It is that if your gut, made up of trillions of microbes, suddenly starts to have imbalance and "bad bacteria" are taking over your gut it can eventually lead to host of other diseases. -You must bring your gut flora into balance.

IS CANDIDA BEATING UP YOUR PROBIOTICS?

As we discussed, there are countless symptoms that arise from the imbalance in your gut. One of the biggest culprits is overgrowth of candida. If you suffer from candida, you may have following symptoms:

Oral Thrush

White patches on your tongue, inner cheeks,

tongue, gums, etc. It may be painful and may hurt during swallowing.

Fibromyalgia/Chronic Exhaustion

This could be due to lack of hydration, minerals, magnesium deficiency or countless other reasons, however if it is tied in with some of the other symptoms, you may want to see the possibility of candida overgrowth.

Digestive Problems

This is very common- you may suffer from IBS, GERD, Constipation, Diarrhea. This could be your imbalance between beneficial bacteria and bad bacteria. Some argue that eventually this will lead to more serious diseases such as ulcerative colitis and Crohn's disease.

UTI Infection

Recurring yeast and UTI infection. Frequent or urgent need to urinate, pain/discomfort in vagina or penis. Some of these symptoms may be tied to bladder and other causes. I'M NOT A DOCTOR AND YOU SHOULD CONSULT A DOCTOR. But I have done excessive research and if you surfer from unexplained bladder or urinary pain or frequent UTI consider checking out *"Bladder And Interstitial Cystitis Pain Holistic IC Diet And Medical Treatment Options For Chronic Pain Relief: Bladder Pain & Urinary Tract Infection Symptoms, Treatments Cure Relief"* book.

CAUSE OF GUT IMBALANCE

In short-It is because today's diet is out of whack!!! Everything you consume has sugar or some form of antibiotics in it, which also kills of the "good bacteria" in your gut. If you look at your milk, meat, even some of the vegetables are all treated with antibiotics. These antibiotics have their purpose to kill off pathogens. However, they also kill of "good bacteria" in your gut, and this symbiotic relationship in your gut has existed for thousands of years. This results in imbalance in your gut, many ailments (including some unexplained symptoms) emerge because you are losing the fight between "good bacteria vs. the bad bacteria."

Most of the time controlling your sugar intake and increasing probiotics in fermented food such as kefir will help in combating candida.

TRUTH IN REBALANCING YOUR GUT

Increase Fermented Foods Intake:

Any fermented food such as sauerkraut, kimchi, yogurt, and my favorite kefir will help! These foods help you because during regular use they help balance your equilibrium between good and bad bacteria in your gut. The reason I like kefir is because you can manipulate what good bacteria you introduce into your drink. I will show you how later.

Avoid/Limit Sugar:

One of the biggest reasons you are losing this fight is because of overconsumption of sugar! Sugar is everywhere! Sugar is even in things that you do not necessarily find sweet, i.e., bread, milk, cheese, etc.... There are other foods that are not sugary but turn into sugar in your gut, such as white flour, refined flour, and other wheat products. Sugar is labeled with terms like "syrup" or "dextrose" or even "sugar alcohol." If the product has sugar alcohol, the manufacturer is not required to report it in nutrition labeling. There are many packages out there that are labeled with only small amount of sugar, but when you eat them, they taste sweet, well they make them sweet by sugar alcohol, and did you know they don't even have to label sugar alcohol in the ingredient list? Sugar alcohol is hidden sugar. It is very hard to know actual consumption when you have hidden sugar like this. Sugar feeds those "bad bacteria, eventually these bacteria cause lots of issues, common symptoms are flatulence, GERD, acidity, burp, etc. But overgrowth of candida can lead to other issues such as bladder problems (rising from yeast, fungi, and bacterial infection).

Avoid Chlorinated Water

Most tap water you drink has chlorine in it- which is a disinfectant. The municipalities have good intention of chlorinating your water so that you do not get sick from pathogens that lurk in the contaminated water; however, chlorine also wipes out the good bacteria in your gut. Therefore, I recommend you buy a filter that removes most of the chlorine. If you like you can also consider purchasing bottled water. However, know that bottled water companies are regulated by......NO ONE! Some of this is a fraud since water is water; there is a famous saying within the water sanitizing industry, all the water you drink was once in someone's toilet-it just recycled! As gross as it sounds, it is probably true.

Take Antibiotic Course Wisely

There is also over prescription of antibiotics. Anytime you go to the doctor because you have a cold and you do not feel great, there is that reliable course of antibiotics that completely wipes out your gut flora. The only thing is you must be on that course for 7-10 days and you will feel great! Guess what; you were going to feel great in 7-10 even without the antibiotics-it called your immune system, and it had nothing to do with the course of antibiotics. Do not get me wrong there are definitely use for antibiotics and your doctor knows best, however I'm making a general assumption that there is over prescription of antibiotics in my opinion and this could be leading to unbalanced gut. The course of antibiotics will wipe out your flora and then you consume food with sugar to exacerbate the problem.

Avoid Meat/Milk Processed with Antibiotics

Maybe you drink chlorine free water, and you have not had dosage of antibiotics in a very long time. In fact, you do not even eat that much sugar, well did you know most of the meat items and milk products are loaded with antibiotics? Milk treated with antibiotics will also make it hard for you to make kefir out of it. The antibiotics and over pasteurizing will denature enzymes that do not allow any good bacteria to thrive. It is important to get good milk as this is the base for kefir. Some people prefer raw milk, but there are also health risks with raw milk, so consider this option wisely.

Interesting how the food industry works, first you

are sold food filled with antibiotics to get you sick and then they sell you all the probiotics to make you better! How convenient a way to make money from both sides! How about we just do not intake the antibiotics in the first place!

With all these ANTI biotics in your gut how will the PRO biotics survive?

I recommend you start consuming fermented food, such as kefir which is loaded with probiotics. However, if you are set on the probiotic you like, I will show you how to introduce your probiotic strain into your kefir, so you do not have to buy the strains ever again! If you are going to introduce a probiotic into your kefir, make sure you get a good probiotic (not necessarily the best marketed or the most expensive). This is an art in itself-what are good probiotics?

CHAPTER 4: HOW TO BUY TOPNOTCH PROBIOTIC PILLS

There are trillions of probiotics in kefir. Most of the bacteria in probiotics are either dead or in dormant stage that needs to be revived again. I highly recommend kefir over purchasing probiotics pills. This is because it is homemade, you can drink organic kefir by buying organic milk, you can manipulate strains in your kefir, you are guaranteed that there are not seas of dead/ineffective/expired bacteria, and it is a lot cheaper! In addition to all of this, you are also obtaining other minerals, vitamins, good fats, amino acids, and antimicrobial agents with kefir.

However, if you are looking to purchase probiotics, here are some recommendations.

There are literally thousands of probiotics out there, which one should you choose?

Well, you should choose the one that works for you. You can get this by trial and error, read independent reviews not the reviews you see on the company's website. Also keep in mind many blogs are actually not independent review. There are hidden links there to bring you over to the company's website, to only sell their products, so be cautious!

GUIDELINES TO PURCHASING PROBIOTICS

Here are some things you should look for in good probiotics.

As I mentioned before looking for probiotics that are straight from the manufacturer, most probiotics die in transit due to lack of refrigeration, storage, etc.

Look for expiration date if they have none you should think about how long they have been sitting on the shelf.

Look to see if they have an enteric coat to make it pass the acids in your stomach.

Ensure you are consuming adequate amount-see the dosage.

Ensure the probiotics are not from fluff companies, try to buy from reputable companies.

Do it straight from the manufacturer. This will prevent mishandling by the third party. Place your order on Sat-Tues so that you can get your order by Friday! You do not want to order on Wednesday through Friday, since this means they may be sitting without refrigeration at some local post office over the weekend before they get to your door. If you order them on Sat-Sun, most likely they will be shipped on Monday. -Tues, they will be ready for shipment and get your order before the weekend. If you are going to pay high price for probiotic capsules, it doesn't make sense to save some money on shipping and have it take 5-7 days for you to get it, since most of the time they are not stored in refrigeration during transit and thus losing its potency and the ones that do come with ice pack, it's barely enough to come in contact with all sides. Most marketers will never tell you this, but it is just a fact!

Do your own research and do not be swayed by marketers, ask the right questions.

INSTEAD, SAVE THOUSANDS OF DOLLARS,

ADD STRAINS OF YOUR CHOICE AND GURANTEE LIVE ORGANIC THRIVING PROBIOTICS IN A DRINK THAT TASTE GOOD BY MAKING YOUR OWN KEFIR.

LET'S GET STARTED!

CHAPTER 5: HOW TO MAKE ULTIMATE KEFIR: STEP BY STEP!

I would advise against buying store bought kefir drinks or making kefir from powdered starter. Kefir made from real grains is delicious, thick, and creamy. You can taste the difference! Kefir made from REAL, LIVE ORGANIC KEFIR GRAINS also has far reaching benefits and you get to control the consistency, flavoring and free from preservatives.

This is a step-by-step guide to make live organic milk kefir. There are many recipe books out there to make all kinds of flavored water kefir. However, this is the foundation of maintaining your live organic strains thriving. You can always add flavoring later (mint, coconut also goes good with flavoring).

Once you buy kefir grains, it goes through transit

and arrives at your house. Your number one challenge will be to ensure the kefir grains stay alive! I have had many consumers who bought kefir from me, complain that they were not able to reproduce kefir because microbes in those grains died! If you have had a hard time having kefir strains stay alive, there could be many reasons that I will discuss as well.

Once you get your kefir grains, please do not get frustrated, give yourself some time and patience.

EQUIPMENT NEEDED

I would also consider making kefir from fresh raw organic milk; however, I am able to make kefir fine with pasteurized milk. I would stay away from ultra-pasteurized milk. Pasteurizing kills off ALL (good and bad) bacteria, thus making it harder for the beneficial bacteria to revive later in the process.

Also, please do not use any metallic utensils, this includes metal spoons--for some reason kefir grains do not produce good results with metallic objects.

<u>EQUIPMENTS:</u>

- ✓ 2 Glass jars preferred, or you can use glass with a wide surface area-do not use glass that is tall and narrow.

- ✓ Plastic strainer

- ✓ Plastic or wooden spoon

- ✓ Paper towel/cloth or coffee filter, which is breathable.

Ingredients

You have two basic and obvious ingredients here:

<u>Whole milk</u> – Do not use ultra-pasteurized milk or

lactose free milk (lactose is needed during fermentation). Raw organic milk is ideal. However, as mentioned, keep in mind the benefits as well as the risk of using raw milk. When the milk goes through pasteurization it kills good and bad bacteria, denatures some of the enzymes.

You can use 2% but stay away from nonfat milk. Goat milk is ok as well. You can try Organic, full cream Jersey cow milk.

Almond milk and coconut milk may be fine for taste and blending, but not in replicating your grains, there is no lactose in them-so you will not use this to reproduce your grains but only as an additive. Have the milk ready before you get the grains, even if you do not have the best milk, dump them in milk as soon as you get them. Your grains need lactose as a food source. They have been shipped to you, sometimes in adverse weather conditions.

Kefir grains- You will need one packet or about 1 tablespoon of good quality kefir grains. Organic ones are always recommended-know your source! Kefir grains are replicated so there may not be a "better" strain, but if you have multiple strains, it may increase your chance of combating an ailment (same reason you purchase probiotics with different strains).

Things to look for in good quality kefir grains:

✓ Multiple kefir grains (different strains) in a batch are a plus. My grains are purchased from various vendors and then I have mixed them all together to form one batch. This allows for various strains to co-exist and gives me greater effectiveness.

✓ The medium they use to produce kefir. I.e., Raw, or organic grass-fed milk in production.

✓ Proper handling and managing - Cross contamination of utensils, debris, improper handling with hands, etc. This could lead to dull kefir grains that may not be thriving.

Quality of grains matter, so initially get the grains from a reputable source. However, if your grains are growing, they can ferment and have probiotics in them.

Important Notes

✓ Wash your hands before starting out!

✓ Do not use metal, ideally use glass or plastic and wood.

✓ Do not use chlorine water or tap water (unless filtered, blended, and chance to aerate)

✓ Never use hot water

✓ Leave kefir out at room temperature for optimal growth (Must be between 70-100F.)

✓ Key is the right amount of milk and right amount of time.

✓ Do not use microwave to heat up kefir, milk, or water.

✓ Do not place in direct sunlight.

STEP-BY-STEP GUIDE

Once you get the grains and have everything lined up, follow these steps to ensure the best probiotic experience and to see health results multiply fast!!!

Revitalize the grains after delivery time. They may take a few days to get going.

Step 1:

Take the grains out of the bag and place them into the jar IMMEDIATELY. Do this right away, not tomorrow, not in the evening but as soon as you get these grains. Why? Because they have been in shipment, they have been surviving without lactose and mostly rough environment. You do not want these grains to die off, that will be a waste of your money. At least dump them in a glass of milk if nothing else for now. Leave the milk at room temperature, not in refrigeration. Refrigeration will slow down your production.

If you want organic kefir, make sure to use organic whole milk. Note for some reason it may be harder to make kefir with ultra-pasteurized organic milk, which are commonly found in stores.

Step 2:

When you have time, within the next 12hrs. Strain the grains out, discard the rest of the milk and pour some new milk on it, enough to cover the grains fully with milk but do not waste milk by filling the whole jar or even half the jar, as you are slowly trying to get them accustom to new milk/home and recover from shipping journey and you don't want to waste milk (especially if it's organic or raw milk which is expensive to begin with). The other thing is the kefir grains stick to the bottom; therefore, short wide glass is preferable to long tall glass. This will maximize the surface area. If you get time, also stir, or VERY GENTLY shake the jar, this allows for new fresh milk (full of lactose) to encounter the grain. This also prevents your grain from becoming brownish color, this brown color with film is the formation of yeast and acetobacter colonies. Ideally it would be best to have constant agitator (nonmetallic).

Step 3:

Cover the jar or glass with paper towel or cloth and rubber band it to the neck of the jar/glass. Make sure you do not cover the jar/glass tightly with lid- kefir grains need oxygen also carbonation could explode your bottle. Grains also need some air circulation.

-Leave them in this milk for few hours (3-5hrs). Avoid sunlight.

-Strain the kefir grains and place them in the jar

again, (You can discard the milk).

-THIS TIME: Fill in twice as much milk (1/4 fill for 500 ml jar) in the jar/glass and gently stir the milk and kefir grains and this time leave them in the jar 7-8hrs, you can gently stir every few hours...it is highly recommended but not mandatory.

Step 4:

Follow step 1-3 again.

Step 5:

BUT NOW: Fill the Jar half full and leave them for 12hrs-remembering to gently stir every few hours.

Step 6:

Follow steps 1-3 again.

Step 7:

FINALLY: Fill the Jar full-leave 1-2 inches from the

rim and leave the kefir grains for 24 hours-
Remember to stir every few hours.

Step 8:

Strain Kefir grains and collect milk/kefir into another glass. Take a spoon and taste the milk/kefir if milk tastes like rotten milk do not consume and follow steps 1-3.

Step 9:

You can repeat the cycle now by just filling the kefir grains with 3/4 to full Jar of kefir every 24hours.

It may take some repetition and tasting your kefir to know how you like it. Ideal milk kefir is a little tart, little fizz to it, creamy and not full separation. Other than that, it is really how you like it. I like to add soda stream and mix my kefir half/half (remember no chlorine in the water).

Troubleshooting Tips

Why do I see physical separation between white liquid and clear liquid?

If you start to see a physical separation where the white liquid separates from the clear liquid that is an indication that you are leaving the kefir grains in there too long OR you need to add more milk. Another word means lactose has been converted and there is no more lactose left for your strains.

YUK! Why is my drink so sour!

Remember lactose is sugar that is needed for your live strains. When sugar is gone, and fermentation occurs the sweetness goes away. If your kefir is too sour, you are either leaving it in there too long or there is very little milk and too many grains.

My milk tastes rotten, why?

Some complain about rotten milk when the fermentation is not completed! Given enough time for fermentation to complete. Milk should not taste rotten, if you feel you have given enough time, throw away the milk and add fresh milk again.

The consistency and taste vary by preference. However, kefir should be a little thicker than milk, not sweet but slightly sour and has a little fizz to it!

Once you have mastered this you are good to go! Enjoy a glass of kefir every day!!! Remember to strain the grains and place them into new whole milk every 24hrs. Ultimately you will find the grains striving and you will have more grains which reach your desire outcome at faster rate. You may produce kefir drink within 12hrs and not 24hrs and you will see your kefir grow. At this time, you have the option to store additional kefir or start to make larger batches.

REMEMBER THE TRICK IS TO GET THE RIGHT AMOUNT OF MILK, THE RIGHT AMOUNT OF TIME AND RIGHT AMOUNT OF KEFIR. BE SURE TO FOLLOW THE CORRECT PROCEDURE DESCRIBED ABOVE. AS MENTIONED, MOST OF THE TIME YOU ARE NOT GETTING GREAT KEFIR IS BECAUSE OF THE PROCESS NOT THE GRAINS! DON'T WASTE MONEY ON BUYING MORE KEFIR GRAINS, FOCUS ON FOLLOWING THE PROCESS.

ADDING DIFFERENT STRAINS TO YOUR KEFIR

Kefir grains are naturally full of probiotics, so even though you may not see improvement over night, you should see changes over time. If you have been using probiotics pills that have been working marvelously for you but are now making the switch to kefir read on!

Your gut is made up of trillions of probiotics, some help you and some are parasites. There are vast number of probiotics out there. Did you know with kefir you can cultivate your own strains?

Kefir has many beneficial strains. Obviously, it does not have ALL the strains out there.

Let us say after much research you have bought your perfect probiotics and it has been helping you or you research a company that has specific strain that know other probiotic company has. Now you can incorporate that strain into your kefir, here is how:

Make sure you buy capsule form of the strain you

want to cultivate.

Step 1:

Once you have made your kefir from kefir grains, take half of it, and save it!

Step 2:

Once you are ready to ferment new kefir or add milk/water to your grain add the content of your favorite capsule on top of the grains and add milk/water.

Step 3:

Remember the strains are competing with one another, so there are three scenarios:

-New strain (probiotic) that you just introduced into kefir to ferment may outcompete and replace the kefir grain. Probiotic strain will replicate and pretty much you are now drinking kefir full of your probiotic that you bought from the stores for FREE!

-New strains will co-exist with kefir strains; this is the ideal situation, now you will get the benefits of kefir strains and the new probiotic strains all in one drink! This is the best scenario!

-New strains will not be allowed to thrive and will eventually die off and the strains in kefir will continue to replicate. In this scenario you are not getting the effects of your new probiotic strains into your kefir. In this case you may want to add more than one capsule into the fermentation process. You may also want to continue to reintroduce capsule after capsule into your fermentation process. It may take a month or so for a new probiotic strain to take over the old strain or find a happy medium where they both co-exist. Once this has happened, you no longer need to buy that particular probiotic EVER AGAIN as that strain has been implemented into your kefir and if it can replicate itself and does not die off.

VACATION – NEED A BREAK

As you continue to do this process, your kefir will start to grow increasingly. At some point in time, you may need a break, but you do not want your kefir grains to die off. You have couple of options at this time:

Slow Down the Growth

You can slow down production by refrigerating the kefir. Place the kefir with milk inside of the refrigerator. What takes a day to produce will now take up to a week to produce! Keep in mind your timing, this may result in foul tasting kefir, refer to above troubleshooting tips.

Stop the Growth

If you are not up for dealing with kefir but plan to use them somewhere down the line, you may want to store them for up to a year! Isolate the grains from the milk, add some dry milk powder, pack them loosely in plastic bag or plastic/glass container (make sure glass does not break and place them inside the freezer. This should buy you some time. When you are ready to revive them, follow the instruction above what you should do when you first get the grains.

CONCLUSION

WHAT TO EXPECT WITH DAILY KEFIR INTAKE

IF it is your gut-balance flora that was causing your ailment, you should see the biggest improvement in your digestion, gas, bloating, constipation, and other gut related symptoms. Other secondary improvements because of optimal gut flora could be to reduce inflammation of the lungs, reduce allergies, less acne, improvement in cholesterol control, reduce in anxiety and depression and increase in energy. All of these are bioproducts of your gut.

Thank you again for your purchase!

I hope you were able to maximize your benefit from healthy probiotics.

PLEASE LEAVE A QUICK 2 SENTENCE REVIEW-
WHAT YOU HAVE TO SAY MATTERS MORE
THAN YOU THINK!